Your Guide
to
Child
Obesity

Elisabeth Holberg, MPH

Table of Contents

Introduction

I have a master of public health degree, a bachelor of science degree in dietetics, and associate of science degree in child development.

My goal for this book is to make child obesity simple for everyone to understand. I also hope that this book helps you maintain a healthy weight by providing information on nutrition and physical activity, and helpful tips. I hope you enjoy this book and I hope it has a positive impact on your life and the lives of the kids you know!

What is Child Obesity?

Child obesity is one of the biggest health concerns facing the United States.

What is obesity?

Obesity means having an excess amount of body fat (NIDDKD, 2012).

Adult BMI (age 20+)	
18.4 or less	Underweight
18.5-24.9	Healthy weight
25-29.9	Overweight
30 or higher	Obese

What is BMI?

BMI stands for body mass index. It is used to determine if you are overweight or obese. BMI is calculated by taking your weight in pounds divided by your height in inches squared. This number is then multiplied by 704.5. It can also be calculated by dividing your weight in kilograms by your height in meters squared.

What does it mean to be at or above the 95th percentile?

If a child is at or above the 95th percentile than five percent of children their age weigh more than them and 95% weigh less than them.
What is the definition of child obesity?

Child obesity is determined using the 2000 Centers for Disease Control and Prevention growth charts (Yanovski, 2005). These charts provide age- and sex- specific standards for children between ages two and twenty (Yanovski, 2005). They are included later in this book. Children who place in the 95th percentile or higher, for BMI, are considered obese (Yanovski, 2015). Children who place between the 85th and 94.99th percentile, for BMI, are considered overweight (Yanovski, 2015). Weight for length and head circumference charts are used for children from birth to age 3; they are also found later in this book.

How common was obesity and child obesity in 2016?

35.1% of American adults over the age of 20 are obese (CDC, 2016). 20.5% of children between 12 and 19 years old are obese (CDC, 2016). 17.7% of children aged six to eleven are obese. 8.4% of two to five-year-old children are obese (CDC, 2016).

How have child obesity rates changed since the 1960s?

Child BMI rates were stable between the 1960s and 1980s and then rose until the 2000s (Von Hippel & Nahhas, 2013). The Fels Longitudinal Study found that BMI distribution was fairly normal for children born from the 1930s until the 1970s (Von Hippel & Nahhas, 2013). Women during this time had an earlier rise in overweight status than their male counterparts (Von Hippel & Nahhas, 2013).

What are the effects of obesity?

Obese children are more likely to become obese adults.

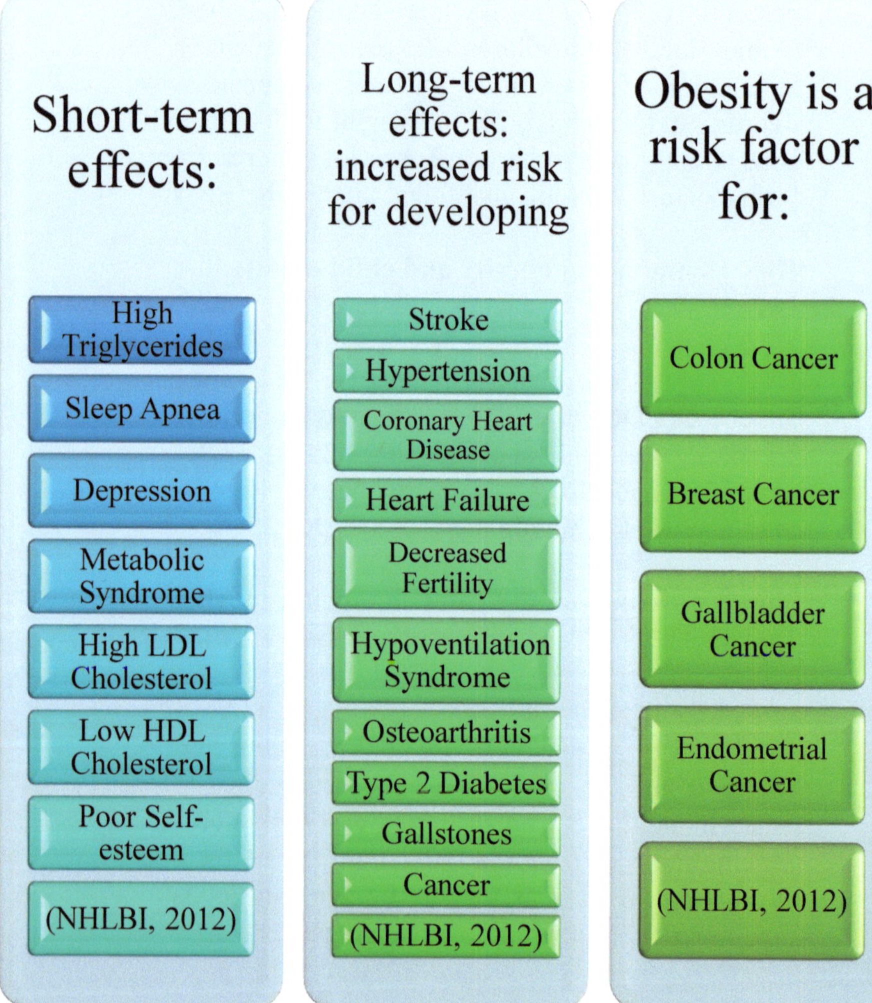

What Factors Affect Child Obesity?

How does obesity affect different racial groups?

Between 2011 and 2014 African American adults had the highest prevalence of obesity compared to all other racial groups in the United States; they were followed by Hispanics then non-Hispanic whites (CDC, 2015). From 2011 to 2014, Hispanic children had the highest rates, followed by non-Hispanic blacks, then non-Hispanic whites, and then non-Hispanic Asians (CDC, 2017).

How does wealth or socioeconomic status affect obesity?

Children from low socioeconomic status families are the most likely to be obese while children from affluent families are the least likely to be obese (Mccaig, 2012). This is likely because poor families have less access to healthy foods and information about nutrition (Mccaig, 2012).

What factors influence obesity?

Individual Level

- Genetics, epigenetics, education, stress, access to healthy food and information about nutrition, diet, food preferences, habits, self-esteem, body image and various life events such as pregnancy or getting divorced (Kahan et al., 2014).

Interpersonal Level

- A person's work environment, having family and friends who are obese, following a poor diet, and living a sedentary lifestyle (Kahan et al., 2014).

Structural and Community Factors

- The culture of the community and access to health care (Kahan et al., 2014).

Social and Policy Factors

- The price and availability of healthy and unhealthy foods, advertising, and which crops are produced (Kahan et al., 2014).

What factors influence child obesity?

- Metabolism,
- Short sleep duration,
- Diet,
- Physical activity level,
- Genetics, and
- Community safety and neighborhood design (CDC, 2018).

How does living in a rural (country) vs. urban (city) area affect obesity rates?

People living in rural populations are more likely to be obese than people living in urban populations (Befort, Nazir & Perri, 2012). 39.6% of adults in rural regions are obese compared to 33.4% urban populations (Befort et al., 2012). People in rural populations consume more calories from fat and have less access to healthy foods (Befort et al., 2012).

How Can Child Obesity Be Prevented?

How do you lose weight?

Weight loss requires being active and eating well. If you want to lose weight then you need to burn more calories than you consume (CDC, 2015). Healthy weight loss is one to two pounds per week. If an adult wants to lose one pound of fat, he or she needs to burn 3500 calories. If you burn an extra 500 calories a day, then you should lose one pound per week (CDC, 2015).

What is the difference between kcals and calories?

Calories refer to energy. Kcals or kilocalories is the unit used to measure calories.

What are some strategies for losing weight?

- Eat a healthy and balanced diet,
- Be more active,
- Pay attention to what you eat and your activity level,
- Eat slowly,
- Do not finish your food if you are not hungry,
- Give your metabolism a boost by eating breakfast and exercising,
- Avoid eating dessert every day,

⊞ Eat at a dinner table instead of in front of the TV,

⊞ Avoid eating out of a container; portion out your food instead,

⊞ Eat smaller portions, and

⊞ Choose water instead of sugar-sweetened beverages (CDC, 2015).

What can parents do to help their children maintain a healthy weight?

- ✓ Balance the calories children consume from their food with the calories they burn through growth and physical activity.
- ✓ Provide healthy foods:
  - o Whole-grain products.
  - o Fruit and vegetables, ideally fresh or frozen.
  - o Low-fat or non-fat milk or dairy products.
  - o Lean protein (poultry, fish, beans, meat, and lentils).
- ✓ Avoid serving large portions.
- ✓ Encourage your children to drink water.
- ✓ Limit sugar, saturated fat, and sugar-sweetened drinks.
- ✓ Make a few small, easily achievable changes at a time.
- ✓ Try to make recipes healthier by replacing ingredients with healthier (less salt, less fat, and less sugar) ingredients.
- ✓ Limit the presence of high-calorie foods at home.

- ✓ Provide fresh fruit and vegetables as snacks, instead of sweet, salty, or high-fat snacks.
- ✓ Be active with your kids (walk, dance, play outside, visit a gym or wellness center, play sports, stretch, or just move).
- ✓ Limit screen time (tablets, video games, TV, computer, and phone) to a maximum of two hours per day.
- ✓ Reduce sedentary behaviors (move as much as possible).
- ✓ Avoid letting children under the age of two watch TV.
- ✓ (CDC, 2017).

What are some other suggestions?

- ⌘ Model good behaviors.
- ⌘ Be active and eat well as a family.
- ⌘ Talk to your doctor about normal growth and development.
- ⌘ Talk to your doctor about maintaining a healthy weight.
- ⌘ Find and use community resources like parks, community centers, wellness centers, your local health department, the internet, social media, libraries, and more.

What is my opinion on weight loss?

I believe it is easy on paper because if you can burn more calories than you consume you should lose weight. However, when you start considering the variety of factors affecting obesity it becomes more complex. It also requires commitment and long-term lifestyle changes. People often get stuck in yo-yo dieting because they lose weight quickly, return to their old habits, and gain the weight back. Remember healthy weight loss is only one to two pounds per week. Also remember that fad diets do not usually work, long term.

My advice:

- ☆ Keep it simple. I love throwing a fresh fruit or vegetable like an apple or a bag of carrots into my lunch bag. I eat yogurt almost every day for breakfast; it is cheap, easy, and provides a lot of healthy bacteria, as well as some calcium and protein. I love putting whole-wheat rice in my rice cooker for an easy and healthy meal.
- ☆ Visit thrift stores to find cheap kitchen items and exercise equipment.
- ☆ Pack your own lunch for work so you do not have to eat fast food or go to a restaurant.
- ☆ Find someone to provide encouragement and accountability such as a family member, friend, co-worker, spouse, partner, or roommate.
- ☆ Make exercise easy and convenient. I have a yoga mat, stair stepper (which cost me less than $80), balance cushion, and exercise ball in my living room. If you get a break at work, you can spend it walking in a hallway or outside.

☆ Make healthy habits part of your routine. If you are consistent, being active will become a habit and you will have to think less about it.

☆ Remember, being active and eating well takes discipline and self-control - but you can do it! Find something that works for you and stick with it.

☆ If you can, visit a community center or gym and participate in exercise classes. You can buy an exercise DVD, or find an exercise class online.

☆ I cook in advance and enjoy the convenience of eating leftovers. You can also prepare extra quantities of ingredients, to be used for meals later in the week.

☆ Have fun with whatever you do.

Nutrition Basics

What should you do about fruits?

- Remember that fruit and juice are high in sugar.
- Choose 100% juice.
- Limit juice consumption to one cup per day.
- Add water to juice to make it less sweet.
- Buy fruit canned in its own fruit juice.
- Fresh fruit (in season) is the healthiest, followed by frozen, then canned.

What should you do about vegetables?

- Fresh vegetables (in season) are the healthiest, followed by frozen, then canned.
- Buy vegetables canned in water, or labeled low-salt.

What should you do about grains?

- Choose grains labeled whole wheat or whole grain. These contain all three parts of the grain (bran, germ, and endosperm). The bran and germ have most of the nutrients. They are removed during processing and must be added again. Items not labeled whole wheat or whole grain do not have all three parts of the grain.

What should you do about dairy and protein?
- Choose low-fat or fat-free items.

Physical Activity

How much physical activity do you need?

- ⚽ Children age 6-17 years old: at least 1 hour per day.
    - ⚾ Aerobic (walking quickly, running, or any exercise that raises your heart rate): at least 3 days each week.
    - ⚾ Muscle strengthening (stretching, climbing, gymnastics, or push-ups): at least 3 days each week.
    - ⚾ Bone strengthening (jump rope, jumping, running, or more): at least 3 days each week.
- ⚽ Adults age 18-64 years old: 2.5 hours each week of moderate intensity aerobic activity (walking quickly, gardening, water aerobics, ballroom dancing, and more) and muscle strengthening activities at least twice a week OR 1 hour and 15 minutes each week of vigorous intensity aerobic activity (running, aerobic dancing, jumping rope, hiking, jogging, and more) and muscle strengthening activities at least twice a week.
- ⚽ (CDC, 2015).

Serving Size

What is one serving for adults?

- 1 teaspoon of butter or margarine (1 dice).
- 3 ounces of meat (1 deck of cards).
- 1 cup of pasta (baseball).
- 1.5 ounces of cheese (4 stacked dice).
- ½ cup of fresh fruit (1 tennis ball).
- (Denny, 2015).

What is one serving for children?

- 1 ounce or slice of bread (1 cd cover).
- 1 ounce or cup of dry cereal (1 baseball).
- 1 small fruit (1 tennis ball).
- 1 cup of vegetables (1 baseball).
- 1 cup of milk or yogurt (1 baseball).
- 1.5 ounces of cheese (1 9-volt battery).
- ½ cup of ice cream (1/2 a baseball).
- 3 ounces of meat (1 deck of cards).
- (Shield & Mullen, 2017).

Supplements

Given my educational background, I am biased against supplements for the average person. The recommendations for how much of a nutrient you should consume (RDAs and DRIs) are a bell curve so you may need more or less than the recommendation. All vitamins except A, D, E, and K will leave the body in your urine when you consume too much. Therefore, Americans have the most expensive pee in the world (Americans, in general, load their bodies up with excess vitamins and minerals they do not need). Vitamins A, D, E, and K leave the body through fat in your stool. Also, the body is very good at reusing nutrients so you are less likely to lose a vitamin you need.

I recommend athletes, pregnant women, people with serious illness, and the elderly take more regular supplements. For everyone else, who can get their nutrients from their food, take a multivitamin a few times a week. This should ensure your body is getting what it needs. Remember many supplements may be a placebo so you think you feel differently, but in fact this is due to your expectation that you will feel different. If you can purchase and preparing your own food you should not need to replace a meal with a supplement drink. I have no objection to giving children a children's vitamin to ensure they have the nutrients they need for proper development. Always talk to your doctor before beginning a supplement program.

Interventions

Most interventions for child obesity, you can find are family focused or school based programs. Personally, I like family focused programs because they focus on the family unit making changes together. I think they can be more effective because they help parents create a strong foundation for their children. This book is family focused and my hope is that you can use this book to create a strong foundation of healthy habits for the children in your life. This book should also provide enough information on nutrition and weight loss that it can help you maintain a healthy weight. The downside to family focused interventions are that participation can be a challenge for busy families.

I have studied some great school based programs like Fit Kids 360. School based programs are great because they help kids be active and learn about the importance of healthy eating and physical activity. They are easy to implement because they require little effort from parents and they occur while children are at school. The downside is that children can engage in a positive environment at school and then go home to a less positive environment.

Food Labels

Read food labels. Remember that one package may contain multiple portions. Pay special attention to calories, salt, sugar, and fat. The percent daily value gives you an estimate of how much of each nutrient the food has, compared to how much you should eat each day.

Nutrients

Fat		
Fatty Acid	**Source**	**Function**
Linoleic fatty acid (omega 6 fatty acid)	Plant oils.	They increase inflammation.
Linolenic fatty acid (omega 3 fatty acid)	Seed oils, fish, walnuts, flaxseed, fish oil, and canola oil.	They decrease inflammation, blood clots, triglycerides and blood pressure. They lower LDL cholesterol and may raise HDL cholesterol, but won't lower it (this is good). They can thin the blood if taken in excess.
Stearic fatty acid	Chocolate.	Polyunsaturated fatty acid.
Oleic fatty acid	Olive oil.	Monounsaturated fatty acid.
Myristic fatty acid	Coconut and palm oils.	Saturated fatty acid.
Monounsaturated fatty acids	Avocado, peanut butter, peanut, olive, and canola oil.	They lower LDL cholesterol and won't lower HDL cholesterol (this is good).
Saturated fatty acids	Animal products.	They lower HDL cholesterol and raise LDL cholesterol (this is bad).
Polyunsaturated fatty acids	Sources include nuts, sunflower seeds, safflower, and sunflower oils.	These lower LDL cholesterol and HDL cholesterol (this is good). Linoleic and linolenic

		fatty acids are polyunsaturated fatty acids.
Trans fat	Fried food and baked goods.	This raises LDL cholesterol and lowers HDL cholesterol (this is bad).

*Remember, you want your HDL cholesterol to be
high and your LDL cholesterol to be low.

Fat Soluble Vitamins		
Vitamin	**Source**	**Function**
A	Egg yolk, butter, whole milk, beef liver, fatty fish, and fish liver oils.	Essential for vision, growth, reproduction, and proper immune function.
Beta carotene	Carrots, red, orange and green veggies, dark green leafy veggies, yellow and orange fruit, cantaloupe, peaches, squash, tomatoes, pumpkin, corn, and peppers.	Beta carotene is an antioxidant that can be converted to vitamin A.
E	Soybean oil, sunflower oil, peanut oil, corn oil, wheat germs, margarine, flaxseed, sunflower seeds, and peanuts.	Antioxidant and protects cell membranes.
D	Egg yolk, butter, fortified milk, anchovies, red and pink salmon, shrimp, tuna, cat fish, and fortified soy milk or rice milk. It	Helps raise calcium in blood when it is low, blood

	can be made in your body from cholesterol.	pressure regulation, immune function, hormone production, and nervous system function.
K	Broccoli, cabbage, spinach, green tea, kale, chick peas, lentils, beans, canola oil, and soybean oil.	Blood clotting and bone health.

Water Soluble Vitamins		
Vitamin	**Source**	**Function**
Thiamin/B1:	Whole and enriched grains, pork, sunflower seeds, and legumes.	Essential for metabolism, and plays a role in nerve conduction.
Riboflavin/B2	Milk, yogurt, whole and enriched grains, pork, beef, squids, clams, eggs, and mushrooms.	Red blood cell formation, digestion, and growth.
Niacin/B3	Whole and enriched grains, liver, tuna, red meat, poultry, mushrooms, and peanut butter.	Helps regulate insulin, digestion, cholesterol production, and nervous system function.
Pantothenic acid:	Plant food, beef, and chicken.	Metabolism, digestion, nervous system function, and hormone production.

Biotin	Eggs, liver, peanuts, cauliflower, most foods but fruit and meat, and some made by bacteria in the intestine	Part of enzymes; used for metabolism.
Folate/Folic acid	Liver, citrus fruit, orange juice, leafy veggies, asparagus, brewer's yeast, chickpeas, garbanzo beans, enriched bread, and cereal.	Cell division, DNA production, metabolism, and birth defect prevention.
B6	Bananas, navy beans, walnuts, beef, potato, salmon, and poultry.	Helps with metabolism and helps produce serotonin.
B12	Animal products.	Assists the nervous system, digestion, and red blood cell formation.
C	Kale, strawberry, rose hips, cantaloupe, citrus fruit, red and green pepper, tomato, and potato.	Prevents scurvy, assists development of cartilage, bone and teeth; plays a role in wound healing, tissue formation and maintenance; helps with immunity; antioxidant.

Minerals		
Mineral	**Source**	**Function**
Magnesium	Almonds, beans, brown rice, coffee, tea, cocoa, whole grains, nuts, peanuts,	Helps with metabolism, influences over 300

	seafood, and green leafy veggies.	enzymes, and helps release insulin.
Iron	Heme sources: meat, poultry, and fish (easier to absorb). Non heme sources: legumes, dry fruit, molasses, green leafy veggies, enriched bread.	Allows transport of oxygen to tissues, allows transport of electrons, immunity, wound healing, and reproduction.
Zinc	Beef, some in chicken and pork, oysters, whole grains, and leafy greens.	Carbohydrate metabolism, needed for insulin response, helps your eyes, needed for breathing, for DNA, RNA and protein synthesis, growth, immunity, and bone and skin integrity.
Copper:	Varies with soil, liver and organ meats, shellfish, nuts, legumes, whole grains, cocoa, and breastmilk.	Antioxidant, nervous system function, bone formation, digestion, and iron metabolism.
Selenium	Nuts, fish, couscous, sunflower seeds, and whole grains.	Helps with immune function and metabolism, antioxidant, reproduction, thyroid function, and can compensate for lack of vitamin E.

| Chromium | Mushrooms, prunes, nits, asparagus, wine, beer, meat, whole grains, and cheese. | Need it for insulin to work correctly and metabolism. |

Macrominerals (you need a lot more of these)

Mineral	Source	Function
Calcium	Dairy, fortified soy, tofu, mustard seed, green leafy veggies, clams, oysters, sardines, almonds, sesame seeds, and molasses.	Mineralization of bones and teeth, nerve function, blood clotting, and stimulation of secretions, cardiac, and skeletal muscle.
Phosphorous	Cheese, beef, chicken, legumes, yogurt, tofu, milk, and sunflower seeds.	Bone formation, helps with metabolism, and part of DNA and RNA.

Electrolytes

Electrolyte	Source	Function
Sodium	Salt, salty or smoked meat, pickled foods, canned soups or veggies, bouillon, MSG, soy sauce, cheese, milk, bread, and potato chips.	Helps with water/pH balance, nerve transmission, and muscle contraction.
Chloride	Salt.	Maintains pH, part of hydrochloric acid, and needed for enzyme activation.
Potassium	Heart function, growth and development, nervous	Banana, avocado, raisins, orange

	system function, muscle contraction, and helps with water/ pH balance and cell membrane transfer.	juice, dairy, cantaloupe, potato, peaches, and tomato.
Iodine:	Soil, salt water, and iodized salt.	Helps body maintain basal metabolic rate (burning calories), reproduction, thyroid hormone production, and growth and development.
Fluorine:	Fluoridated water.	Mineralization of bones and teeth.
Manganese:	Whole grains, cereals, fruits, nuts, veggies, tea, wine, and instant coffee.	Bone formation, wound healing, and metabolism.
Molybdenum:	Plant foods (depending on soil).	Required for intrauterine and postnatal development.

Ultra-trace elements (you need very little of these)		
Element	**Source**	**Function**
Arsenic	Water, rocks, soil, pesticides, coal power plants, aerosols, fish, oysters, grains, dairy, and meat.	Formation and utilization of a methyl group.
Boron	Raisins, legumes, nuts, avocados,	Embryogenesis, bone development, cell membrane stability,

	plants, beer, wine, cider, water, antacids, antibiotics, lipstick, and lotion.	mediation of the inflammatory response, and decrease blood glucose.
Nickel	Nuts, legumes, grains, chocolate, and plants (depends on the soil).	Plants- cofactor for enzymes.
Silicon	Plants, water, whole grains, and root veggies.	Promote bone growth and collagen formation.
Vanadium	Black pepper, parsley, dill weed, mushroom, shellfish, grains, and sweeteners.	Mimics insulin.
Cobalt	B12	Part of vitamin B12.

Menus

* All menus are taken from the U.S. Department of
Health and Human Services National Institute of
Health National Heart, Lung and Blood Institute.

American Cuisine: 1200 calories (NHLBI, n.d.)

Breakfast				
Food	Energy (Kcal)	Fat (GM)	%Fat	Exchange for:
Whole-wheat bread, 1 med. slice	70	1.2	15	(1 Bread/Starch)
Jelly, regular, 2 tsp	30	0	0	(½ Fruit)
Cereal, shredded wheat, ½ C	104	1	4	(1 Bread/Starch)
Milk, 1%, 1 C	102	3	23	(1 Milk)
Orange juice, ¾ C	78	0	0	(1½ Fruit)
Coffee, regular, 1 C	5	0	0	(Free)
Breakfast Total	389	5.2	10	

Lunch				
Food	Energy (Kcal)	Fat (GM)	%Fat	Exchange for:
Roast beef sandwich Whole-wheat bread, 2 med. slices	139	2.4	15	(2 Bread/Starch)
Lean roast beef, unseasoned, 2oz	60	1.5	23	(2 Lean Protein)
Lettuce, 1 leaf	1	0	0	
Tomato, 3 med. slices	10	0	0	(1 Vegetable)
Mayonnaise, low-calorie, 1 tsp	15	1.7	96	(1/3 Fat)
Apple, 1 med.	80	0	0	(1 Fruit)
Water, 1 C	0	0	0	(Free)
Lunch Total	305	5.6	16	

Dinner				
Food	Energy (Kcal)	Fat (GM)	%Fat	Exchange for:
Salmon, 2 oz.	103	5	40	(2 Lean Protein)
Vegetable oil, 1½ tsp	60	7	100	(1½ Fat)
Baked potato, ¾ med.	100	0	0	(1 Bread/Starch)
Margarine, 1 tsp	34	4	100	(1 Fat)
Green beans, seasoned with margarine, ½ C	52	2	4	(1 Vegetable) (½ Fat)
Carrots, seasoned	35	2	0	(1 Vegetable)
White dinner roll, 1 small	70	2	26	(1 Bread/Starch)
Iced tea, unsweetened, 1 C	0	0	0	(Free)
Water, 2 C	0	0	0	(Free)
Dinner Total	454	20	39	

Snack				
Food	Energy (Kcal)	Fat (GM)	%Fat	Exchange for:
Popcorn, 2½ C	69	0	0	(1 Bread/Starch)
Margarine, ¾ tsp	30	3	100	(¾ Fat)

Daily Total						
Energy (Kcal)	Fat (GM)	%Fat	SFA, % kcals:	Total Carb, % kcals:	Cholesterol, mg:	Salt. mg:
1,247	34	24	7	58	96	1,043

American Cuisine: 1600 calories (NHLBI, n.d.)

Breakfast				
Food	Energy (Kcal)	Fat (GM)	%Fat	Exchange for:
Whole-wheat bread, 1 med. Slice	70	1.2	15	(1 Bread/Starch)
Jelly, regular, 2 tsp	30	0	0	(½ Fruit)
Cereal, shredded wheat, ½ C	104	1	4	(1 Bread/Starch)
Milk, 1%, 1 C	102	3	23	(1 Milk)
Orange juice, ¾ C	78	0	0	(1½ Fruit)
Coffee, regular, 1 C	5	0	0	(Free)
Milk, 1%, 1 oz.	13	0.03	23	(⅛ Milk)
Breakfast Total	402	5.23	12	

Lunch				
Food	Energy (Kcal)	Fat (GM)	%Fat	Exchange for:
Roast beef sandwich				
Whole-wheat bread, 2 med. Slices	139	2.4	15	(2 Bread/Starch)
Lean roast beef, unseasoned, 2 oz.	60	1.5	23	(2 Lean Protein)
American cheese, low-fat and low-	46	1.8	36	(1 Lean Protein)

Food	Energy (Kcal)	Fat (GM)	%Fat	Exchange for:
sodium, 1 slice (¾ oz.)				
Lettuce, 1 leaf	1	0	0	
Tomato, 3 med. slices	10	0	0	(1 Vegetable)
Mayonnaise, low-calorie, 2 tsp	30	3.3	99	(⅔ Fat)
Apple, 1 med.	80	0	0	(1 Fruit)
Water, 1 C	0	0	0	(Free)
Lunch Total	**366**	**9**	**22**	

Dinner				
Food	Energy (Kcal)	Fat (GM)	%Fat	Exchange for:
Salmon, 3 oz	155	7	40	(3 Lean Protein)
Vegetable oil, 1½ tsp	60	7	100	(1½ Fat)
Baked potato, ¾ med.	100	0	0	(1 Bread/Starch)
Margarine, 1 tsp	34	4	100	(1 Fat)
Green beans, seasoned with margarine, ½ C	52	2	4	(1 Vegetable) (½ Fat)
Carrots, seasoned with margarine, ½ C	52	2	4	(1 Vegetable) (½ Fat)
White dinner roll, 1 med.	80	3	33	(1 Bread/Starch)
Ice milk, ½ C	92	3	28	(½ Fat)
Iced tea, unsweetened, 1 C	0	0	0	(Free)
Water, 2 C	0	0	0	(Free)
Dinner Total	**625**	**28**	**40**	

Snack				
Food	Energy (Kcal)	Fat (GM)	%Fat	Exchange for:
Popcorn, 2½ C	69	0	0	(1 Bread/Starch)
Margarine, 1½ tsp	51	6	100	(1½ Fat)
Grand Total	**1,490**	**48**	**29**	

Daily Total						
Energy (Kcal)	SFA, % kcals:	Total Carb, % kcals:	Cholesterol, mg:	Total Fat, % kcals:	Protein, % kcals:	Sodium, mg:
1,490	8	52	142	29	19	1341

Asian- American Cuisine (NHLBI, n.d.)

Breakfast	1,600 Calories	1,200 Calories
Banana	1 small	1 small
Whole-wheat bread	2 slices	1 slice
Margarine	1 tsp	1 tsp
Orange juice	¾ C	¾ C
Milk, 1%, low-fat	¾ C	¾ C

Lunch	1,600 Calories	1,200 Calories
Beef noodle soup, canned, low-sodium	½ C	½ C
Chinese noodle and beef salad		
Beef roast	3 oz.	2 oz.
Peanut oil	1½ tsp	1 tsp
Soy sauce, low-sodium	1 tsp	1 tsp
Carrots	½ C	½ C
Zucchini	½ C	½ C
Onion	¼ C	¼ C
Chinese noodles, soft-type	¼ C	¼ C
Apple	1 med.	1 med.
Tea, unsweetened	1 C	1 C

Dinner	1,600 Calories	1,200 Calories
Pork stir-fry with vegetables		
Pork cutlet	2 oz.	2 oz.
Peanut oil	1 tsp	1 tsp
Soy sauce, low-sodium	1 tsp	1 tsp
Broccoli	½ C	½ C
Carrots	1 C	½ C
Mushrooms	¼ C	½ C
Steamed brown rice	1 C	½ C
Tea, unsweetened	1 C	1 C

Snack	1,600 Calories	1,200 Calories
Almond cookies	2 cookies	—
Milk, 1%, low-fat	¾ C	¾ C

1,600 Calories		1,200 Calories	
Calories: 1,609		**Calories: 1,220**	
Total Carb, % kcals:	56	Total Carb, % kcals:	55
Total Fat, % kcals:	27	Total Fat, % kcals:	27
Sodium, mg:	1,296	Sodium, mg:	1,043
SFA, % kcals:	8	SFA, % kcals:	8
Cholesterol, mg:	148	Cholesterol, mg:	117
Protein, % kcals:	20	Protein, % kcals:	21

Southern Cuisine (NHLBI, n.d.)

Breakfast	1,600 Calories	1,200 Calories
Oatmeal, prepared with 1% milk, low-fat	½ C	½ C
Milk, 1%, low-fat	½ C	½ C
English muffin	1 med.	—
Cream cheese, light, 18% fat	1 Tbsp.	—
Orange juice	¾ C	½ C
Coffee	1 C	1 C
Milk, 1%, low-fat	1 oz.	1 oz.

Lunch	1,600 Calories	1,200 Calories
Baked chicken, without skin	2 oz.	2 oz.
Vegetable oil	1 tsp	½ tsp
Salad:		
Lettuce	½ C	½ C
Tomato	½ C	½ C
Cucumber	½ C	½ C
Oil and vinegar dressing	2 tsp	1 tsp
Brown rice, seasoned with light margarine	⅓ C	⅓ C
Baking powder biscuit, prepared with vegetable oil	1 small	½ small
Margarine	½ tsp	½ tsp
Water	1 C	1 C

Dinner	1,600 Calories	1,200 Calories
Lean roast beef	3 oz.	2 oz.
Onion	¼ C	¼ C
Beef gravy, water-based	1 Tbsp.	1 Tbsp.
Turnip greens, seasoned with	½ C	½ C
light margarine	½ tsp	½ tsp
Sweet potato, baked	1 small	1 small
Light margarine	½ tsp	¼ tsp
Ground cinnamon	1 tsp	1 tsp
Brown sugar	1 tsp	1 tsp
Cornbread prepared with light margarine	½ med. slice	½ med. slice
Honeydew melon	¼ med.	⅛ med.
Iced tea, sweetened with sugar	1 C	1 C

Snack	1,600 Calories	1,200 Calories
Saltine crackers, unsalted tops	4 crackers	4 crackers
Mozzarella cheese, part-skim, low-sodium	1 oz.	1 oz.

1,600 Calories		1,200 Calories	
Calories: 1,653		**Calories: 1,225**	
Total Carb, %		Total Carb, %	
kcals:	53	kcals:	50
Total Fat, % kcals:	28	Total Fat, % kcals:	31
Sodium, mg:	1,231	Sodium, mg:	867
SFA, % kcals:	8	SFA, % kcals:	9
Cholesterol, mg:	172	Cholesterol, mg:	142
Protein, % kcals:	20	Protein, % kcals:	21

Mexican-American Cuisine (NHLBI, n.d.)

Breakfast	1,600 Calories	1,200 Calories
Cantaloupe	1 C	½ C
Farina, prepared with 1% milk, low-fat	½ C	½ C
White bread	1 slice	1 slice
Margarine	1 tsp	1 tsp
Jelly	1 tsp	1 tsp
Orange juice	1½ C	¾ C
Milk, 1%, low-fat	½ C	½ C

Lunch	1,600 Calories	1,200 Calories
Beef enchilada		
Tortilla, corn	2 tortillas	2 tortillas
Lean roast beef	2½ oz.	2 oz.
Vegetable oil	⅔ tsp	⅔ tsp
Onion	1 Tbsp.	1 Tbsp.
Tomato	4 Tbsp.	4 Tbsp.
Lettuce	½ C	½ C
Chili peppers	2 tsp	2 tsp
Refried beans, prepared with vegetable oil	¼ C	¼ C
Carrots	5 sticks	5 sticks
Celery	6 sticks	6 sticks
Milk, 1%, low-fat	½ C	—

Dinner	1,600 Calories	1,200 Calories
Chicken taco		
Tortilla, corn	1 tortilla	1 tortilla
Chicken breast, without skin	2 oz.	1 oz.
Vegetable oil	⅔ tsp	⅔ tsp
Cheddar cheese, low-fat and low-sodium	1 oz.	½ oz.
Guacamole	2 Tbsp.	1 Tbsp.
Salsa	1 Tbsp.	1 Tbsp.
Corn, seasoned with margarine	½ C	½ C
Spanish rice without meat, seasoned with margarine	½ C	½ C
Banana	1 large	½ large
Coffee	1 C	1 C
Milk, 1%, low-fat	1 oz.	1 oz.

1,600 Calories		1,200 Calories	
Calories: 1,638		**Calories: 1,239**	
Total Carb, %		Total Carb, %	
kcals:	56	kcals:	58
Total Fat, %		Total Fat, %	
kcals:	27	kcals:	26
Sodium, mg:	1,616	Sodium, mg:	1,364
SFA, % kcals:	9	SFA, % kcals:	8
Cholesterol, mg:	143	Cholesterol, mg:	91
Protein, % kcals:	20	Protein, % kcals:	19

Lacto-Ovo Vegetarian Cuisine (NHLBI, n.d.)

Breakfast	1,600 Calories	1,200 Calories
Orange	1 med.	1 med.
Pancakes, made with 1% milk, low-fat and egg whites	(3) 4" circles	(2) 4" circles
Pancake syrup	2 Tbsp.	1 Tbsp.
Light margarine	1½ tsp	1½ tsp
Milk, 1%, low-fat	1 C	½ C
Coffee	1 C	1 C
Milk, 1%, low-fat	1 oz.	1 oz.

Lunch	1,600 Calories	1,200 Calories
Vegetable soup, low-sodium, canned	1 C	½ C
Bagel	1 med.	½ med.
Processed American cheese, low-fat and low-sodium	¾ oz.	—
Spinach salad		
Spinach	1 C	1 C
Mushrooms	⅛ C	⅛ C
Salad dressing, regular calorie	2 tsp	2 tsp
Apple	1 med.	1 med.
Iced tea, unsweetened	1 C	1 C

Dinner	1,600 Calories	1,200 Calories
Omelet		
Egg whites	4 large eggs	4 large eggs
Green pepper	2 Tbsp.	2 Tbsp.
Onion	2 Tbsp.	2 Tbsp.
Mozzarella cheese, made from part-skim milk, low-sodium	1½ oz.	1 oz.
Vegetable oil	1 Tbsp.	½ Tbsp.
Brown rice, seasoned with ½ tsp light margarine	½ C	½ C
Carrots, seasoned with ½ tsp light margarine	½ C	½ C
Whole-wheat bread	1 slice	1 slice
Light margarine	1 tsp	1 tsp
Fig bar cookie	1 bar	1 bar
Tea	1 C	1 C
Honey	1 tsp	1 tsp

Snack	1,600 Calories	1,200 Calories
Milk, 1%, low-fat	¾ C	¾ C

1,600 Calories		1,200 Calories	
Calories: 1,650		**Calories: 1,205**	
Total Carb, %		Total Carb, %	
kcals:	56	kcals:	60
Total Fat, %		Total Fat, %	
kcals:	27	kcals:	25
Sodium, mg:	1,829	Sodium, mg:	1,335
SFA, % kcals:	8	SFA, % kcals:	7
Cholesterol, mg:	82	Cholesterol, mg:	44
Protein, % kcals:	19	Protein, % kcals:	18

Age/Weight Charts

*All charts are taken from the Center for Disease Control and Prevention, National Center for Health Statistics

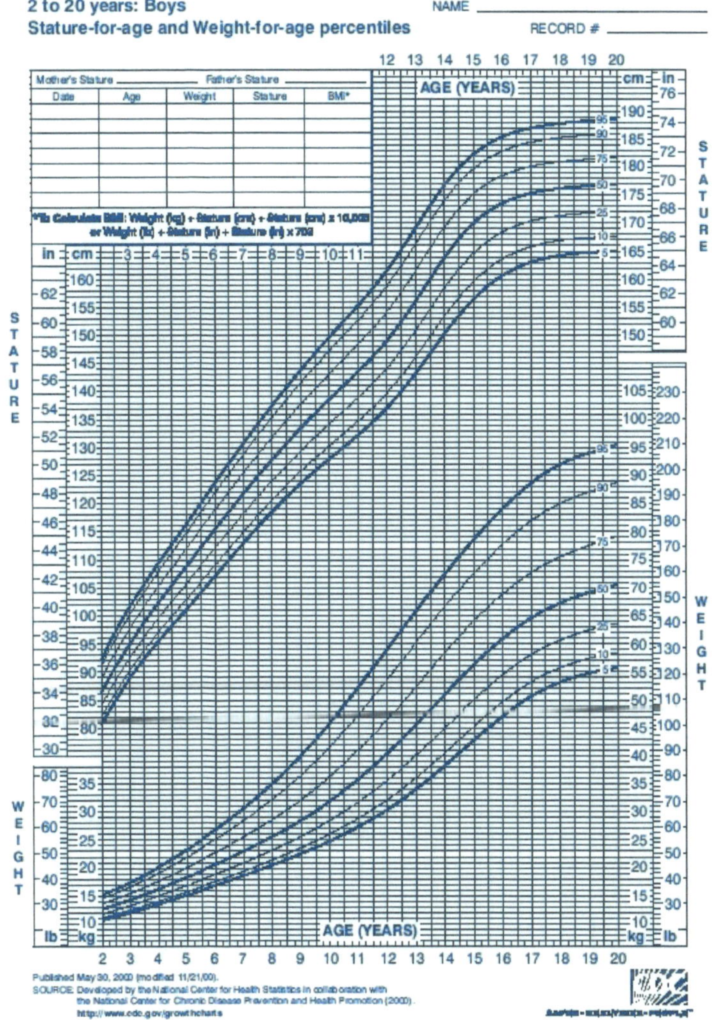

(CDC, 2017)

2 to 20 years: Boys
Body mass index-for-age percentiles

NAME ___________________________

RECORD # ___________________

Date	Age	Weight	Stature	BMI*	Comments

*To Calculate BMI: Weight (kg) ÷ Stature (cm) ÷ Stature (cm) x 10,000
or Weight (lb) ÷ Stature (in) ÷ Stature (in) x 703

Published May 30, 2000 (modified 10/16/00).

SOURCE: Developed by the National Center for Health Statistics in collaboration with
the National Center for Chronic Disease Prevention and Health Promotion (2000).
http://www.cdc.gov/growthcharts

SAFER · HEALTHIER · PEOPLE

(CDC, 2017)

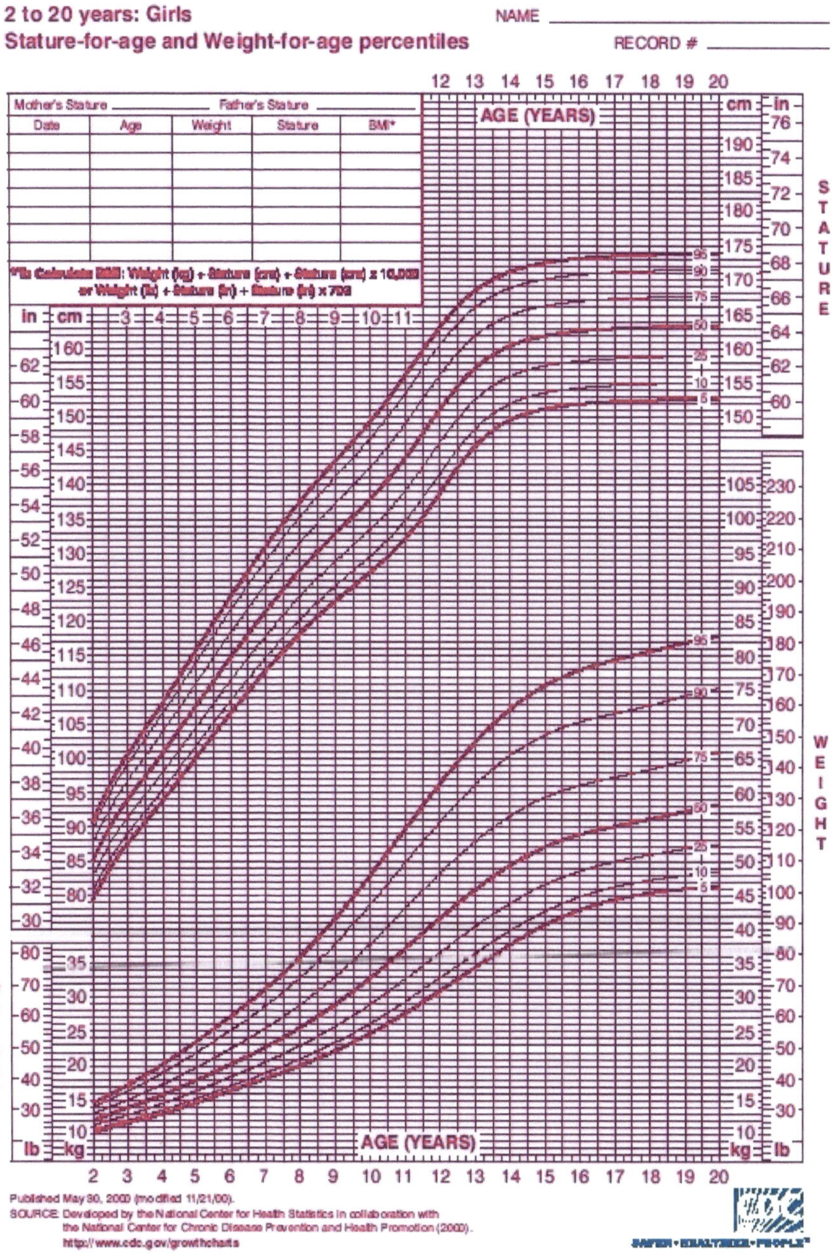

2 to 20 years: Girls
Stature-for-age and Weight-for-age percentiles

NAME ________________________

RECORD # ________________________

(CDC, 2017)

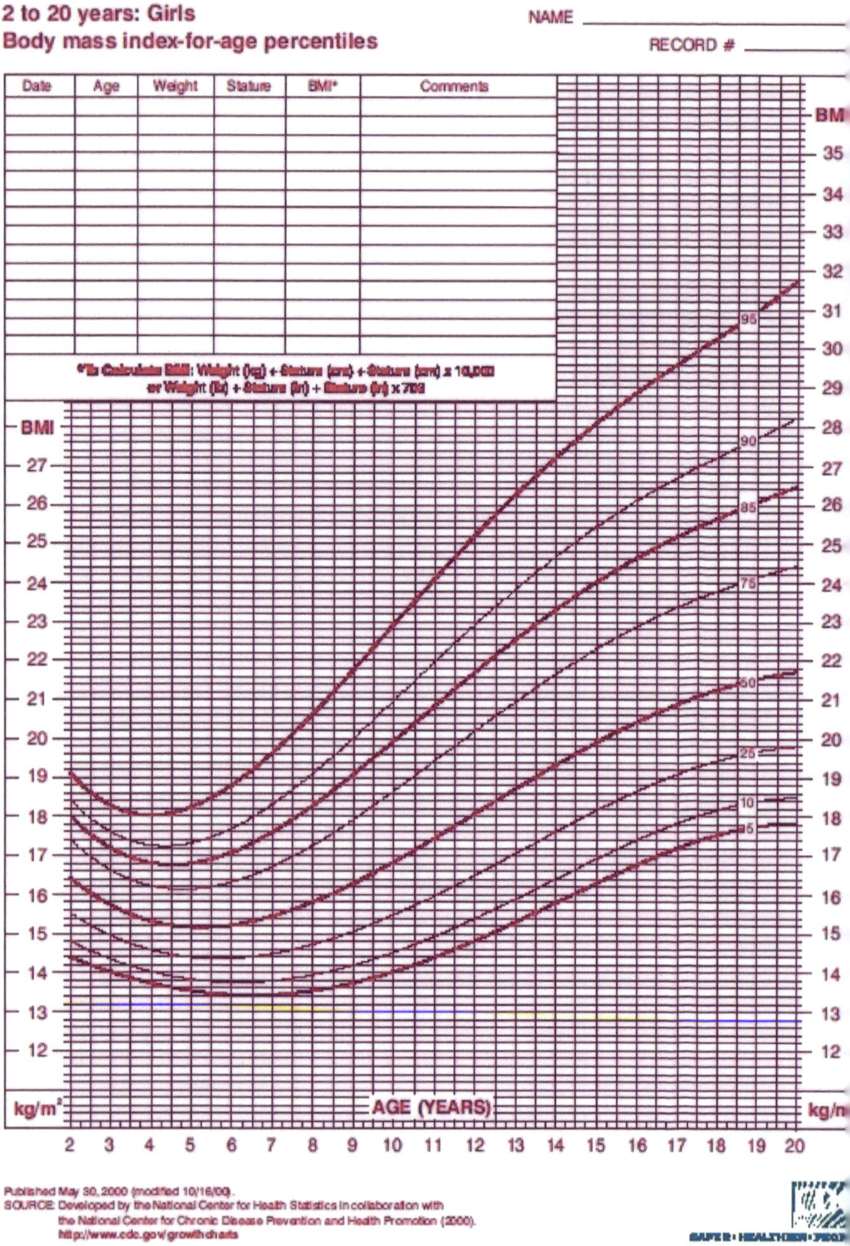

2 to 20 years: Girls
Body mass index-for-age percentiles

NAME ___________________

RECORD # ___________________

Date	Age	Weight	Stature	BMI*	Comments

*To Calculate BMI: Weight (kg) ÷ Stature (cm) ÷ Stature (cm) x 10,000
or Weight (lb) ÷ Stature (in) ÷ Stature (in) x 703

AGE (YEARS)

kg/m²

Published May 30, 2000 (modified 10/16/00).
SOURCE: Developed by the National Center for Health Statistics in collaboration with
the National Center for Chronic Disease Prevention and Health Promotion (2000).
http://www.cdc.gov/growthcharts

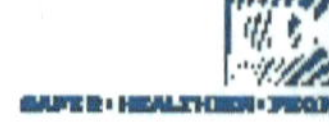

(CDC, 2017)

Birth to 36 months: Boys
Head circumference-for-age and
Weight-for-length percentiles
NAME
RECORD #
AGE (MONTHS)
Birth   3   6   9   12   15   18   21   24   27   30   33   36
HEAD CIRCUMFERENCE
WEIGHT
LENGTH
Date   Age   Weight   Length   Head Circ.   Comment
Published May 30, 2000 (modified 10/16/00).
SOURCE: Developed by the National Center for Health Statistics in collaboration with
the National Center for Chronic Disease Prevention and Health Promotion (2000).
http://www.cdc.gov/growthcharts

SAFER · HEALTHIER · PEOPLE

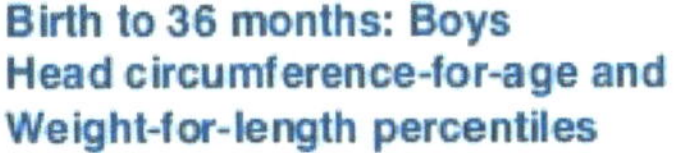

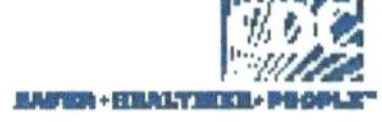

(CDC, 2017)

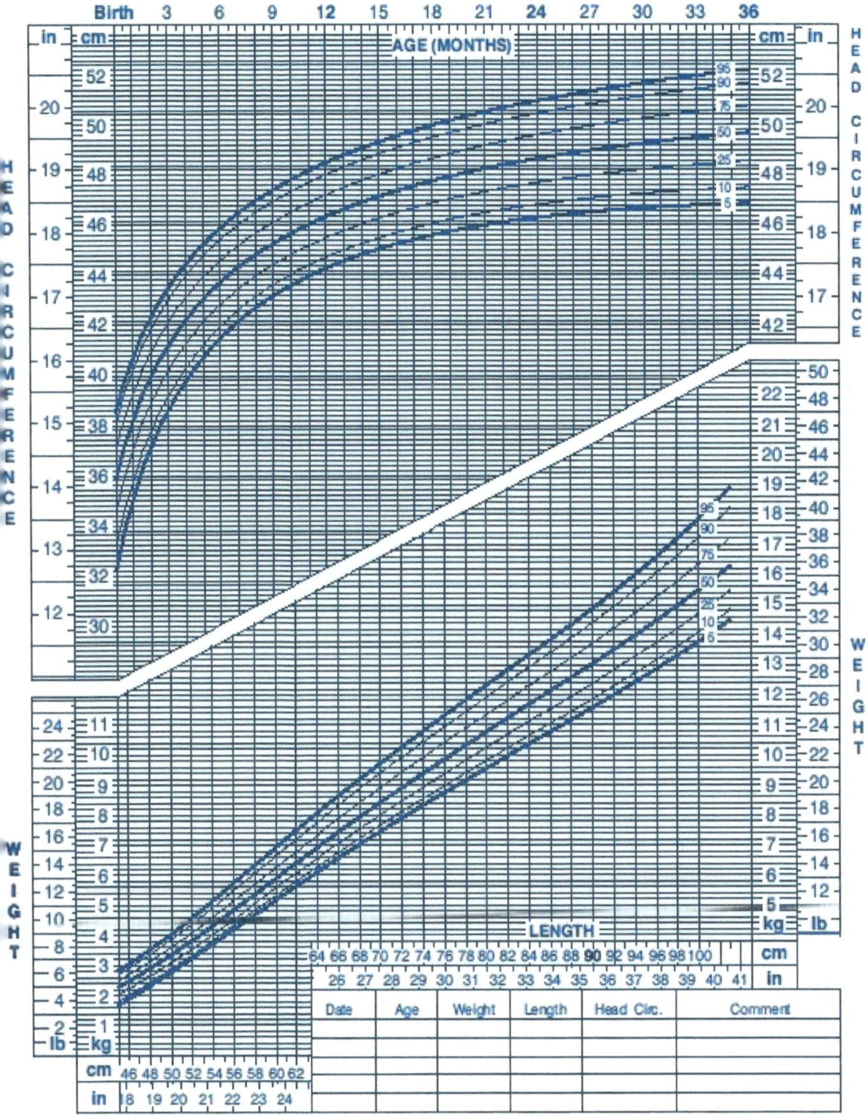

Birth to 36 months: Boys
Length-for-age and Weight-for-age percentiles

NAME _______________

RECORD # _______________

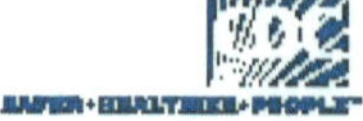

(CDC, 2017)

Birth to 36 months: Girls
Length-for-age and Weight-for-age percentiles
NAME
RECORD #
AGE (MONTHS)
Birth 3 6 9 12 15 18 21 24 27 30 33 36
in cm
LENGTH
cm in
WEIGHT
AGE (MONTHS)
12 15 18 21 24 27 30 33 36
Mother's Stature
Father's Stature
Gestational Age: Weeks
Comment
Date Age Weight Length Head Circ.
Birth
Birth 3 6 9
Published May 30, 2000 (modified 4/20/01).
SOURCE: Developed by the National Center for Health Statistics in collaboration with
the National Center for Chronic Disease Prevention and Health Promotion (2000).
http://www.cdc.gov/growthcharts

SAFER · HEALTHIER · PEOPLE™

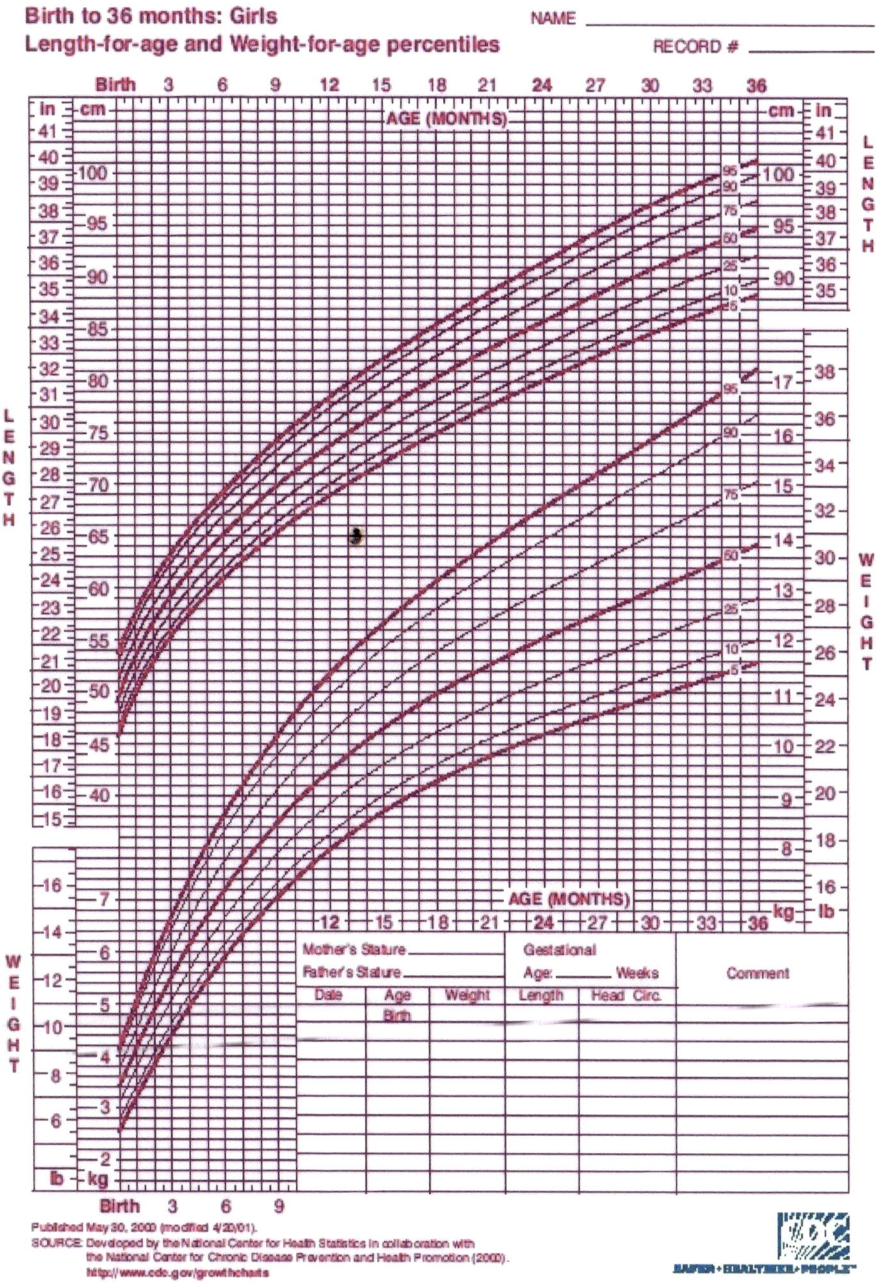

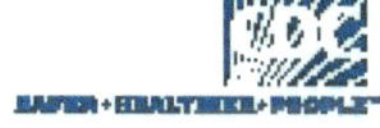

(CDC, 2017)

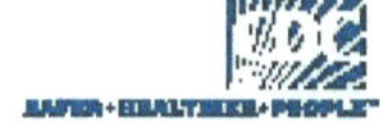

(CDC, 2017)

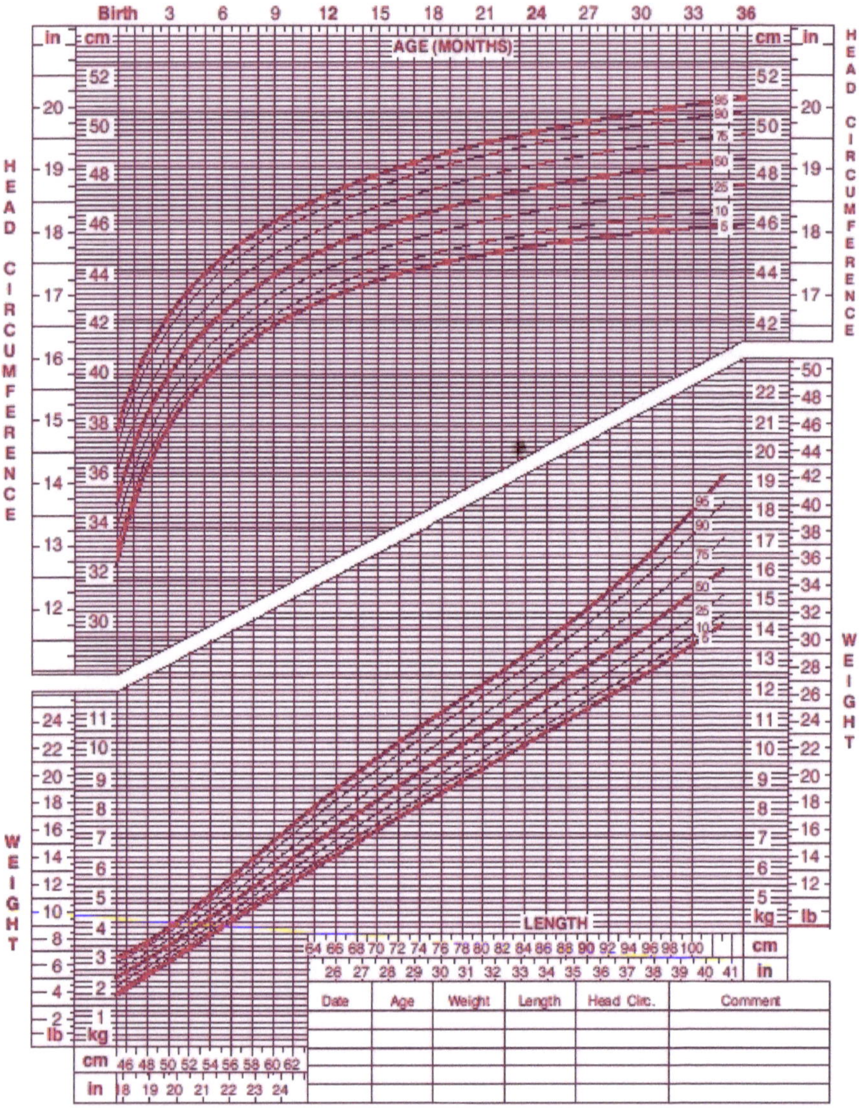

References

Befort, C. A., Nazir, N., & Perri, M. G. (2012). *Prevalence of obesity among adults from rural and urban Areas of the United States: Findings from NHANES (2005–2008)*. The Journal of Rural Health: Official Journal of the American Rural Health Association and the National Rural Health Care Association, 28(4), 392–397.http://doi.org/10.1111/j.1748-0361.2012.00411.x

CDC. (2015, May 15). *Healthy weight.* Retrieved from https://www.cdc.gov/healthyweight/index.html

CDC. (2015, June 4). *Physical activity basics.* Retrieved from https://www.cdc.gov/physicalactivity/basics/index.htm

CDC. (2015, September 11). *Obesity prevalence maps.* Retrieved from http://www.cdc.gov/obesity/data/prevalence-maps.html

CDC. (2016, February 25). *Obesity and overweight.* Retrieved from http://www.cdc.gov/nchs/fastats/obesity-overweight.htm

CDC. (2017, April 10). *Childhood obesity facts.* Retrieved from https://www.cdc.gov/obesity/data/childhood.html

CDC. (2017, September 13). *Tips for parents – Ideas to help children and maintain a healthy*

weight. Retrieved from
https://www.cdc.gov/healthyweight/children/
index.html

CDC. (2018, January 29). *Child obesity facts.*
Retrieved from
https://www.cdc.gov/healthyschools/obesity/f
acts.htm

Denny, S. (2015, March 20). *Serving size vs. portion
size: Is there a difference*. Retrieved from
http://www.eatright.org/resource/food/nutriti
on/nutrition-facts-and-food-labels/serving-
size-vs-portion-size-is-there-a-difference

Kahan, S., Gielen, A.C., Fagan, P. J., & Green, L.
W. (Eds.). (2014). *Health behavior change in
populations.* Baltimore, MD: Johns Hopkins
University Press.

Mccaig, Amy. (2012, November 9). *Childhood
obesity more likely to affect children in
poorer neighborhoods*. Retrieved from
http://news.rice.edu/2012/11/09/childhood-
obesity-more-likely-to-affect-children-in-
poorer-neighborhoods-according-to-new-
rice-study/

NIH: NHLBI. (2012, July 13). *What are the health
risks of overweight and obesity*? Retrieved
from http://www.nhlbi.nih.gov/health/health-
topics/topics/obe/risks

NIH:NHLBI. (n.d.). *Menus.* Retrieved from
https://www.nhlbi.nih.gov/health/educational
/lose_wt/eat/menus.htm

NIH: NIDDKD. (2012, October). Overweight and
Obesity Statistics. Retrieved from
http://www.niddk.nih.gov/health-

information/health-
statistics/Pages/overweight-obesity-
statistics.aspx

Shield, J.E. & Mullen, M. (2017, March 15). *Kids
and portion control*. Retrieved from
https://www.eatright.org/food/nutrition/dietar
y-guidelines-and-myplate/kids-and-portion-
control

Von Hippel, P., & Nahhas, R. (2013). *Extending the
history of child obesity in the United States:
The fels longitudinal study, birth years 1930-
1993*. Obesity, 21(10), 2153-2156.

Yanovski, J. (2015). *Pediatric obesity*. An
introduction. Appetite, Appetite.

www.ingramcontent.com/pod-product-compliance
Lightning Source LLC
Chambersburg PA
CBHW040235240726
48664CB00001B/146